Prepper Parents!

*A Beginner's Guide to Surviving
Societal Meltdown & Mayhem with your Family*

Prepper Parents!

*A Beginner's Guide to Surviving
Societal Meltdown & Mayhem with your Family*

Ma & Pa American

Black Lyon Publishing, LLC

PREPPER PARENTS!
Surviving Society Meltdown and Mayhem with your Family
Copyright © 2013 by Ma & Pa American

All rights reserved. No part of this book may be used or reproduced in any way by any means without the written permission of the publisher, except in the case of brief quotations embodied in critical articles and reviews.

Please note that if you have purchased this book without a cover or in any way marked as an advance reading copy, you have purchased a stolen item, and neither the author nor the publisher has been compensated for their work.

Our books may be ordered through your local bookstore or by visiting the publisher:

BlackLyonPublishing.com

Black Lyon Publishing, LLC
PO Box 567
Baker City, OR 97814

ISBN-10:   1-934912-56-5
ISBN-13: 978-1-934912-56-0

Written, published and printed in
the United States of America.

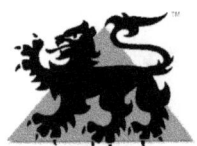

Black Lyon
NONFICTION

Contents

Introduction 1

The Plan 2

The Go-Bag 4

Water 11

Food 14

Heat, Cooking, Shelter and Light 19

Defense 22

Medical and Dental 25

Personal Hygiene 30

Finance and Bartering 32

Communication 35

Hunting, Fishing and Gardening 37

Power and Transportation 41

Above and Beyond 43

Introduction

"Failing to plan is planning to fail." —Benjamin Franklin

All over this great country of ours, millions of people are quietly, behind-the-scenes, preparing for disaster like they've never prepared before. No two preppers or survivalists are alike. No two will prepare the same. No two have the same resources. But all have the same goal: survival.

Preparing to survive on your own can seem overwhelming at first. It doesn't have to. We've heard some people claim if you're only starting to prep now, you're too far behind to catch up. Don't believe a word of it!

This manual is intended to be a brief, easy, no-nonsense kind of book focused on protecting the people under your own roof should doom and gloom actually strike. As parents, our thoughts are first and foremost about the wellbeing of our family. The universe revolves around our little ones. And we have to keep ourselves safe in order to keep *them* safe.

You might ask what's different now? Why the sudden interest in TV shows and manuals? Earthquakes, hurricanes, tornadoes and floods haven't increased exponentially. Though most prepping serves double-duty to help us as Americans prepare for natural disasters, many of us are far more concerned about the impact our ever-expanding government, its spending and stifling regulations will have on us as citizens in the near future. We look to the future and see the potential for economic collapse, martial law, and societal breakdown like never before. We hope for the best but prepare for the worst.

The Plan

Prepping is no longer on the fringe. With TV shows dedicated to the subject, doomsday prepping has become mainstream. But to do it right, you need a plan.

Remember how in school as a child you planned for fires, earthquakes and so on? So if a fire broke out in school or in your home, ideally you didn't even have to pause and think. You didn't panic. You knew what to do.

☑ **ACTION ITEM:**   *Decide to make a plan!*

Parents need to plan.

And parents need to keep their plans quiet. Secret even. Only those intimately involved with your survival plan need to know what you're doing, what you have stored, how much you're spending, where you're going and so on.

• TIP: Keep your plan quiet!

It might seem counterintuitive, but very young children in your household don't need to know the details of the plan. They only need to know if mommy or daddy says they're going to do The Plan, they need to do exactly what they're told because it's super important. That's all. Any other details may accidentally get repeated to other kids at school, and those kids' friends or parents in return. So much for secret! The older your children get, the more you can fill them in.

It's also important not to obsess. You're trying to prepare, not control the universe. Also, how much sense does it make to throw away the quality of the life you have today because you're always worrying about tomorrow? Take your family vacations! Go on romantic dates! Don't become so frenzied in your prepping that your children become frightened. Preparations are your responsibilities as parents. Let your little ones be carefree little ones while they can. Enjoy your own life until and unless it's time to change.

☑ ACTION ITEM: *Decide if you'll "bug out" or stay.*

Civilization is only a few days without food away from total uprising. In case of martial law, foreign invasion, the U.S. government turning on its own citizens—or whatever other scenario you equate with the "zombie apocalypse"—eventually you could be targeted for what you have. Stores will run out of food. Potable water will be in short supply, particularly in cities. Heat and electricity may not exist. The needs of your family will be up to you to provide. Depending on your resources, you'll have to choose your safest bet and work out the details of your plan around that location. Here are your options:

- Stay in your home.
- Retreat to the home of a friend or family member.
- Retreat to another bug-out location such as a bunker or shelter.
- Head for the wilderness.

• TIP: Rural areas will generally be safer than urban areas.

☑ ACTION ITEM: *Decide a budget for supplies.*

If you've decided to bolt, you'll need a go-bag stocked for enough days worth of supplies to get you to your planned location. You will also need to stock your home and/or secondary location with enough supplies to survive for a good long while whether you bug-in or have another living space in mind. We'll get into checklists and details for supplies later. For now, just decide how much money you can spend per week or per month.

The Go-Bag

We're tossing the go-bag, a.k.a. bug-out bag prep right here up front. Building your bags is often the simplest and least overwhelming place to start if you're new to prepping. Even if you haven't decided to bug-out as part of The Plan, a stocked bag can also be a good supplement to your home stockpile.

☑ **ACTION ITEM:** *Get online and just look around.*

There are a ton of online stores selling survival gear and supplies. Just Google a few key phrases and you'll find them. You can also peruse places like Cabela's in person. We highly recommend Amazon.com, though. If you have an account, you can simply add any item you see during a search into your shopping cart. You can keep the items indefinitely to purchase later. It doesn't matter if you have hundreds or thousands of dollars worth of supplies in your cart, in the end that cart will essentially become a full list of all the goodies you might want. Then you can buy a little at a time. Amazon also tends to be *cheaper*. Search by "free super-saver shipping" to weed out the vendors that will charge you an arm and a leg to ship a box of waterproof matches.

☑ **ACTION ITEM:** *Decide how many days.*

How far away is your bug-out location? A one-day stroll? A four-day hike? Know this number, and you'll know how many days worth of food, medicine and other supplies you'll need to get in your bag. Go-bags are intended for situations in which you'll have to jump in you car and flee to a second location, or escape on foot. If you find yourself in a situation where you don't need to leave your home, the go-bag contents can still be very useful.

• TIP: Get in shape! Start walking and doing mild weight lifting now.

☑ **ACTION ITEM:** *Buy the bags.*

Don't buy huge, super-expensive hiking or military bags. Just look for an average-sized canvas, water-resistant backpack with multiple zipper pockets. Choose a bag that's black, gray, tan or camo to best blend with your local surroundings. You'll want a backpack, not a duffle or other kind of tote that you'll be stuck swinging over one shoulder or carrying in your hand. Your hands and/or the front of you will need to be free for packing weaponry, holding on to your little ones, and so on.

Teens and pre-teens should be able to handle an adult-sized backpack—just fill it lighter than yours depending on the child's age. Go ahead and buy a small, fun toddler backpack if your kids are walking age. Limit what you put in this bag to a change of clothes and a cherished toy or stuffed animal. Toddlers will feel included this way, but won't be burdened with carrying too much. The toy will also be a comfort. Don't forget to pack a sippy cup.

You will need one go-bag for each member of your family.

For simplicity's sake, we've opted not to address preparedness for your pets. We're focused on you and your children. There are other excellent guides that include chapters on pet prepping already out there on the market.

• TIP: Keep your go-bags as light as possible. 20% of your body weight is a max.

☑ **ACTION ITEM:** *Stock and store the bags.*

It's time to start shopping! Go into your Amazon shopping cart and move some items from the "saved for later" section into the active "cart" section. All it takes is the click of a button. We recommend buying your bag items in order of importance: water, food, heat/shelter, defense, medical supplies and onward.

Bags should be stored in the coolest, darkest place you have available. Freeze-dried emergency or camping foods typically have a shelf-life of more than 10 years. MREs last anywhere from 5-15 years, but if kept in extreme desert heat, have been known to go bad in a year.

While your bags are stored, check them each year and replace anything you feel needs replacing. Nothing goes to waste. Just use the items in your bag and replace them with new items.

• TIP: Keep to your budget. You don't need to fill the bags all at once!

WATER

_____   Personal straw water filter

_____   Water purification tablets

_____   Sealed potable water envelopes

_____   Lightweight aluminum cup (for water and food)

FOOD

_____   Energy/protein bars

_____   Freeze-dried food or MREs with heaters

_____   Small bottle of multi-vitamins

_____ Squeezable fruit/veggie pouches for infants/toddlers

_____ Spork

HEAT AND SHELTER

_____ Waterproof matches

_____ Lighter

_____ Waterproof mylar tent or sleeping bag

_____ Lightweight aluminum pot for campfire cooking

_____ Tinder (a ziplock bag full of dryer lint is light, free and effective)

_____ Shakeable flashlight and/or glowsticks

_____ "Hotties" hand and foot warmers

_____ Travel hatchet

_____ Foldable hiking shovel

DEFENSE AND SECURITY

_____ Handgun or rifle (to be carried separate from the bag)

_____ Ammo

_____ Hunting knife

_____ Duct tape

_____ Para cord

MEDICAL

_____ Band-aids, butterfly bandages, etc.

_____ Antibacterial ointment such as Neosporin

_____ Sanitizing alcohol wipes

_____ Blood clotting pad

_____ Any prescription meds you may need

_____ Extra glasses or contact lenses

_____ Aspirin, acetaminophen, ibuprofen (all three)

HYGIENE AND CLOTHING

_____ Gloves

_____ Socks

_____ Underwear

_____ Cloth feminine napkins

_____ Cloth diapers

_____ Lightweight microfiber towels

_____ Wet wipes

_____ Dry, waterless shampoo, conditioner, body soap

_____ Travel-sized toothbrush, toothpaste, floss

_____ Hairbrush or comb

_____ Travel-size deodorant

The items listed above are just the basics chosen for weight, bulk and necessity. If you have the money, room and physical strength, you may also consider a number of additional items:

MISCELLANEOUS

_____ Foldable campstove and fuel

_____ Battery- or solar-powered radio

_____ Battery-powered lantern

_____ Portable survival fishing kit

_____ Compass

_____ Tampons or disposable pads

_____ Blankets, pillows, bedrolls

_____ Disposable face masks

_____ Razors

_____ Books, playing cards, other entertainment

_____ Emergency dental repair kit

_____ Sewing kit

_____   Sunblock, hat, extra sunglasses

_____   Envelope of your documents such as drivers' licenses,
        birth certificates, credit cards, etc.

_____   Roll of cash and/or ounces of silver or gold if you
        can afford them.

_____   Additional toys and clothing for the kids.

• TIP: Dry, healthy feet are essential for a bug-out.
Band-aids to cover blisters and extra socks are a must.

Water

Alrighty. Now that you have your go-bags, it's time to start thinking about what to do if you've decided to bug-in (stay in your existing location) or move to another house, stronghold, bunker or whatever secondary location you've chosen.

People can go days without food and survive, but will die of dehydration much, much sooner. This fact makes potable water number one on our list of must-haves.

If you're on a municipal water supply, what would happen to you if a major earthquake, hurricane or other natural disaster caused the system to become contaminated? You don't want to be stuck meting out the water in that tea kettle you left on the stove or from the toilet tanks, do you?

• TIP: If you bug out, choose a route and destination near a natural water source.

☑ **ACTION ITEM:** *Store some drinking water.*

First, store some drinking water. Having water is a no-brainer—and we don't just mean a little bit of water. Start with cases of bottled water. Add in a few gallon jugs of water. You can stack these in the garage and leave them for years if need be. Rotate out the cases every couple years to use the oldest and replenish your supply with new water. This will get you by in a pinch.

If you're afraid your location will not be anywhere near a river, creek, well, spring or other fresh water source, you might also consider buying some of those big, blue BPA-free water storage tanks. Survival supply stores all over the internet carry these jugs for just this purpose. They come in five-gallon sizes and up!

☑**ACTION ITEM:** *Prepare three ways to sterilize your drinking water.*

Water gets contaminated in a lot of ways, each of which takes different methods to clean. Bacteria, virus, industrial chemicals, poisons, heavy metals and protozoa are just a few examples. If you're dipping water out of your backyard swimming pool or sipping from the banks of a mountain stream, you may need different ways to clean those water sources.

Water can be cleaned with: portable filters, UV light, chemical tablets or drops, boiling, and steam distilling. That's about it.

- Portable filters will clean most heavy metals and industrial chemicals from water.

- UV light kills parasites, protozoa, viruses and bacteria.

- Chemical tablets or drops such as iodine and bleach pretty much only kill viruses and bacteria.

- Boiling and distilling kills everything, but it will not remove many metals, industrial chemicals, and so forth.

As you can see, you may need to use a combination of methods to get your water clean enough to safely drink. All of the water treatment methods mentioned above are inexpensive for the most part and can be found online or in most camping supply stores.

If you want to go a more expensive route, there are both electric and non-electric water distillers out there on the market, but those can run up to

$500 each. High quality individual water sterilization thermoses are also available for around $175. Personalized water filtration straws will run you less than $20.

It's also a good idea to buy a bag of activated charcoal. Charcoal is "dirt cheap" (ha ha) and lasts almost forever—an excellent way to filter water. Sand can also help filter water when nothing else is available.

- **TIP: Keep plastic buckets or even a big rain barrel on hand to catch rainwater.**

Food

You have to eat. Supermarkets have roughly three days worth of food on their shelves. They rely on daily shipments to be trucked in. But what if a natural disaster has destroyed or blocked the road system? Or martial law has been declared and the government has seized control of food distribution? You're going to need to fend for yourself. The smartest way to go is to stock up on the foods that have the longest shelf life. We're not going to lie—stocking up on food is expensive and takes a long, long time.

• TIP: Store your food in a cool, dark, dry place to extend shelf life.

☑ **ACTION ITEM:** *Start storing foods with long shelf lives.*

Wise Foods and Mountain House are both excellent companies with a wide range of products. A rule of thumb is that any food vacuum sealed and freeze dried in a can is good for 25-30 years. Freeze-dried foods sealed in packages/pouches, plastic bins or mylar envelopes have a 10-15 year average. Canned foods from your grocery store will last 1-2 years. Dry pasta, beans and rice will easily last 10-15 years.

• TIP: Freeze-dried meals sealed in individual pouches pack best in go-bags.

In case of an emergency, use the foods in your refrigerator and freezer first. They will spoil quickest. Next use your supermarket-purchased canned goods, dry cereals, etc. Hit your survival food supply after the easily spoiled foods are gone. You can even mix your survival foods in with supermarket-purchased foods to get the best nutritional value possible. Survival and camping foods contain enough fat and calories to survive on, but they don't contain enough protein, vitamins and minerals to stay healthy long-term. Make sure you have bottle of multivitamins on hand. Liquid vitamins deteriorate in potency the fastest. Chewables and gummies begin to fade the next fastest, followed by capsules. Hard tablets last the longest. You can use vitamins well after their expiration dates. They lose potency and effectiveness, but don't change in their chemical composition in a way that turns toxic.

Below are lists of staples with very long shelf lives.

• **TIP: You WILL need to supplement freeze-dried foods with other foods or vitamins.**

DRY FOODS

_____ Pastas (all varieties)

_____ Beans (all varieties)

_____ Lentils

_____ White rice

_____ White flour

_____ Whole wheat

_____ Yeast

_____ Oats

_____ Corn meal

_____ Granulated (or fresh) honey

_____ Brown sugar

• TIP: Honey NEVER goes bad. Its shelf-life is indefinite!
If honey granulates, heat it to re-liquify.

FREEZE-DRIED, VACUUM-SEALED PACKAGED FOODS

_____ Breakfast meals (varieties)

_____ Lunch meals (varieties)

_____ Dinner meals (varieties)

_____ Desserts (varieties)

_____ Military MREs (with heater)

• TIP: Freeze-dried ice cream and ice cream bars are available.
They last about two years and are great for little kids!

CANNED FREEZE-DRIED/POWDERED FOODS

_____ Butter

_____ Milk

_____ Cheeses

_____ Flour

_____ Salt (iodized)

_____   White sugar

_____   Breakfast meals (varieties)

_____   Lunch meals (varieties)

_____   Dinner meals (varieties)

_____   Desserts (varieties)

_____   Fruits

_____   Vegetables

_____   Meats

_____   Eggs

_____   Crackers

_____   Nuts

_____   Cocoa powder

_____   Pudding powder

_____   Sour cream

_____   Peanut butter

_____   Tomato powder

_____   Onion powder

_____   Soup mixes

- TIP: #10 cans work well for items you'll use quickly. For foods you won't go through as fast, try to purchase in smaller sealed cans to avoid exposing as much food to air.

- TIP: Molasses in glass jars has a shelf life of 25+ years and is an excellent source of iron!

- TIP: Store apple cider vinegar! It's useful as a food, cleaner and much more.

Heat, Cooking, Shelter and Light

Now that you have food and water taken care of, you need to start thinking about the next most important aspect of survival: heat and shelter. Cooking and light are also be tossed into this category as so many of the supplies overlap. If you're bugging-in at your current location, you probably already have a roof over your head, so just heat/cooking/light aspects of this chapter will apply more. Pay attention to the shelter advice if you're planning to drive or hike to a secondary location, and if your secondary location is outdoors. You don't want to prepare this far only to die of exposure.

• TIP: Little ones heat up and cool down faster than adults. Pay close attention!

☑ **ACTION ITEM:**   *Start storing supplies in these categories.*

HEAD AND SHELTER

_____   Waterproof matches—lots of them

_____   Cigarette lighters or click fire starters

_____   Tinder

_____ Kindling

_____ Firewood

_____ Wedge, maul and axe

_____ Chainsaw with extra oil and fuel, chain sharpener

_____ Hand saw

_____ Wool blankets

_____ Heavy clothing

_____ Mylar emergency waterproof blankets and tents

_____ Sleeping bag

_____ Battery-powered fans (for cooling in summer)

LIGHT

_____ Flashlights: battery-powered and shakeable

_____ Glowsticks

_____ Candles

_____ Lanterns: battery powered

_____ Lamps: oil burning, with extra oil

_____ Lightbulbs

COOKING

_____   Pots, bowls, cups, utensils

_____   Propane cook stove

_____   Extra propane canisters

_____   Dutch ovens

_____   Aluminum foil

• TIP: If you don't know what a WakaWaka light is, find out! Same with a Firebox folding camp stove.

Defense

Prepper manuals can get very, very complicated on the subject of defense. Some go even further into offense. We'll try to touch on some basics—things you might need to chase away those trying to steal your supplies or harm your family. You may even have wildlife to defend yourself against depending on whether you're roughing it outside. But let's face it, there are a hundred manuals on the art of war, martial arts, military maneuvers and so on. We recommend looking into one of those books for more in-depth discussion on your personal protection. We're keeping it simple. This is a beginner's guide, after all.

• TIP: Many of the items you'll need for defense will serve double-use for hunting.

☑ **ACTION ITEM:** *Research weapons.*

Each member of your family will ideally need to select and learn how to use a weapon. Even your toddler can learn how to kick an attacker in the shins, bite them or whop them on the nose with a rock. Dad is probably more equipped to pack a rifle or two over his shoulder along with that go-bag. Mom might go for a handgun while your teenager might prefer a knife or bow and arrow. The choice is really about preference, physical ability, proper training and budget. The bigger variety of weaponry available within your family circle, the better.

☑ **ACTION ITEM:**   *Buy a weapon—or ten.*

Here are some of your options. The more variety, the better, but your arsenal will obviously depend on your comfort level using a weapon, skill and budget. Obviously, we're assuming you're using common sense and a well-thought-out approach to safety. You're not going to hand a three-year-old a .38 special.

_____ Hunting rifle

_____ Handgun

_____ Shotgun

_____ Crossbow

_____ Compound long bow

_____ Knife

_____ Bear (pepper) spray

_____ Ammo, arrows, bolts

_____ Slingshot

_____ Baseball bat

_____ Nails (all sizes for repair and self-fashioned weapons)

• TIP: Household items can also make good impromptu weapons. Think: kitchen knife drawers, home office scissors, broom handles, lamp cords ...

☑ **ACTION ITEM:**   *Study basic hand-to-hand combat.*

Take a self-defense class, not just especially if you're a mom. The entire family needs to go. Even if the world doesn't crumble into chaos, it's a very good thing to know how to use your voice, how to defend yourself if attacked, how to fight back, and how to get away unhurt.

For those interested in amping it up a notch, take kick-boxing or martial arts classes. Again, even if you never have to use these skills to defend yourself, your health will thank you.

☑ACTION ITEM: *Get in shape!*

Remember the difference in Sarah Connor from the first *Terminator* movie to the second? Yeah, *that*. Use her as your inspiration! (Okay, we're kidding… a little.) But seriously, start swimming, walking, hiking and lifting a few weights here and there. Do some yoga. Focus on strength, stamina and flexibility. How do you think you're going to escape to your bug-out location four days away if you can't even walk around the block? How are you going to carry a baby, backpack and gun if just carrying in a bag of groceries from the car to the kitchen does you in? Think about it. Your plan is useless if you're physically unable to execute it.

Medical and Dental

Supplies to take care of your medical, dental and vision needs should come next. As parents of little ones, you need these items in your home at all times anyway. Just buy an extra box of Mickey Mouse band-aids here and there, and in no time you'll have the basic medical supplies for your bug-out bag in addition to a well-stocked medicine cabinet.

People without kids aren't going to think about all the separate medications needed. Dose and strength are very different in children's medicine than adult medicine.

Remember, an ounce of prevention is worth a pound of cure. Watch your kids closely. Brush and floss your teeth well. Get regular checkups while you still can. You want to go in to your emergency situation in the best shape you can. Once you're in the middle of the crisis, for the love of God, don't do anything unnecessarily risky. You might not be able to run on down to the E.R. to treat that broken leg or head injury.

☑**ACTION ITEM:** *Put together the mother of all first-aid kits!*

VISION

_____   Extra glasses

_____   Extra contacts

_____ Generic reading glasses (even if you don't need them)

_____ Contact solution

• TIP: Don't ever throw away glasses with your "old" prescription. They may come in useful for someone else, or as bartering items.

DENTAL

_____ Toothbrushes

_____ Dental floss

_____ Toothpaste

_____ Mouthwash

_____ Emergency dental filling kit

_____ Orajel or something similar

MEDICAL

_____ Band-aids (all sizes)

_____ Aspirin

_____ Acetaminophen (Tylenol)

_____ Ibuprofen

_____ Naproxen

_____ Laxatives

_____   Antidiarrheal

_____   Anti-gas medicine

_____   Antibiotic ointment

_____   Antibiotics (penicillin)

_____   Burn gel

_____   Blood clot pad (Quikclot)

_____   Latex sterile gloves

_____   Splints

_____   Slings

_____   Gauze

_____   Butterfly closures

_____   Adhesive tape

_____   Thermometer

_____   Tweezers

_____   Scissors

_____   Eye wash

_____   Snakebite kit

_____   Field surgical instrument kit

_____   Suture kit

_____   Skin stapler

_____   Alcohol sterilizing wipes

_____   Rubbing alcohol

_____   Peroxide

_____   Syrup of ipecac

_____   Antihistamines

_____   Antifungal (such as Tinactin)

_____   Cold medicines

_____   Bag balm (works as vaseline, lotion, and lip balm)

_____   Instant hot packs and ice packs

_____   Icy hot balm

_____   Epsom salts

_____   Sun screen

_____   Bug repellent

_____   Q-tips

_____   Cotton balls/rounds

_____   Potassium iodide (for radiation exposure)

_____   Charcoal tablets

_____   Children's fever reducer with dosage chart

_____   Toddler saline nose spray

_____   Vicks

_____   Children's cough drops

_____   Pediacare drink boxes

_____   Condoms (just sayin'!)

• TIP: If you can't get a prescription antibiotic, fish penicillin is still available online and can be ingested by humans. Doses will need adjusted.

• TIP: Liquid tablets and capsules deteriorate faster and have a shorter shelf life than caplets and tablets.

• TIP: Do not use the antibiotics outside the penicillin family if you don't know much about them. Some antibiotics have a chemical composition that changes rather than becomes weaker, and becomes toxic to humans after the medicine's expiration date.

• TIP: Aspirin is derived from Willow trees. Learn more by researching online about how to make this and other painkillers from the plants, trees, and fungi growing in your area. Aloe vera plants are wonderful to have around to treat minor burns, including sunburns.

Personal Hygiene

Some view the items in this chapter as "luxury" items, only to be bought in large quantities after everything else on your list is completely purchased and stored. The argument is that while you might not enjoy the quality of life you'd have without these items, at least you'd still survive and be alive. We see and understand that point. However, personal hygiene items are not only essential to your comfort—they help fight off disease and poor health. Sanitary is safer. You'll note that some of your personal hygiene items duplicate the items listed in the medical and dental chapter. Makes sense now, doesn't it?

And yes, we also understand that you can use phone book pages and big fuzzy leaves instead of toilet paper when push comes to shove. But why go that route if you don't have to?

• TIP: Soaps and detergents will last for years, but their plastic bottles won't. Transfer these things to glass jars and they'll last ten times longer.

_____   Bar soap

_____   Shampoo

_____   Conditioner

_____   Diapers (both cloth and disposable)

_____ Tampons/feminine pads

_____ Cloth/washable feminine pads

_____ Razors

_____ Extra towels

_____ Toothpaste

_____ Children's fluoride-free toothpaste

_____ Toothbrushes

_____ Dental Floss

_____ Toilet paper (only if you have a large storage area)

_____ Deodorant

_____ Dry, no-rinse body soaps, shampoos and conditioners

_____ Laundry soaps

_____ Bleach

_____ Baby wipes

_____ Hand sanitizer

• TIP: Keep razor blades in a dry place. Blades are dulled more by moisture than by time.

Finance and Bartering

First, the finance part. What we're going to say here might go against everything you've heard before, but bear with us. Do you remember that scene on the movie *Titanic* when the wealthy tycoon tries to buy himself a place on the escape boat? In any survival situation, your money is going to have about the same value as his did—diddly squat. Unless people are in a very well-prepped position themselves, they aren't going to want to trade you for your ounces of gold or silver.

Gold and silver are not items we'd recommend offering for barter. However, they're the items we strongly recommend having for after any long-term crisis such as a complete economic meltdown. (Not so much for a short-term emergency such as floods or earthquakes. Your cash will likely still work fine then.) Jewelry with diamonds and other fine gems may also prove useful.

Silver dollars, half-dollars, quarters, dimes and nickels minted prior to 1965 do contain some amount of silver and will likely still be worth something post-disaster.

All these items are the wealth by which you'll rebuild your finances after the meltdown passes. *Hide this wealth well, and don't let on that you have it—not to anyone.*

☑ **ACTION ITEM:** *Start investing in precious metals. Hide them very, very well.*

A family sitting on a pile of silver as society begins to rebuild will be in a far better position for keeping or obtaining land, a home, a business, etc. than a family with nothing.

> • TIP: Invest in the smallest measurement of precious metals possible. Smaller denominations will be easier to spend.

Starving people will need food. Thirsty people need clean water. People who have just the basics will want just a little bit of luxury, and by luxury we mean the nonessential items they used to enjoy every day before the crisis you prepared for hit.

☑ACTION ITEM: *Start stockpiling barter items.*

The following supplies are excellent to have on hand for trading.

_____ Ground coffee or tea bags (Shelf life of around 2 years if sealed.)

_____ Green coffee beans
(Sealed cans last 30+ years and are easily ground and roasted.)

_____ Tampons and feminine pads

_____ Diapers

_____ Cigarettes, cigars or chewing tobacco

_____ Pain relievers

_____ Salt, pepper and other seasonings

_____ Liquor

_____   Ammo

_____   Matches and lighters

Communication

Don't count on Internet or cell phone service. Don't count on TV, FM radio or even electricity in general for that matter. In a dire emergency, count on chaos and isolation from the news.

> • TIP: If you're bugging out and don't want to be found, leave cell phones and GPSs behind. You can be tracked from these devices.

Your best bet for communicating with the outside world will be a radio. Find a radio that receives FM, AM and shortwave. Shortwave reception is the important feature here. Not only can you find battery-operated radios, but those that are handcrank-powered and solar-powered. Some radios can run on all three of those options. Just remember that you'll be able to hear the news, but you won't be able to transmit news. If you want to be able to communicate, you'll need to look into HAM radio systems. Hearing transmissions is cheap. Making transmissions requires more equipment, training and a much bigger investment all the way around.

☑ **ACTION ITEM:** *Collect a few communication items.*

_____ Short-wave radio

_____ Batteries (all sizes)

_____ Rechargeable batteries (all sizes)

_____   Battery charger (solar and/or electrical)

_____   Rechargeable batteries

And that's all we have to say about that.

• TIP: Solar powered battery chargers do exist. They aren't very expensive either.

Hunting, Fishing and Gardening

You'll need a full set of basic tools for hunting, fishing and gardening. Because of the low nutritional value of long-shelf-life foods, you will always need to supplement them with foods you can kill, cut down, or dig up yourself. It is particularly important for growing children to begin receiving fresh foods to supplement the survival foods as soon as possible.

☑**ACTION ITEM:**   *Gather your tools.*

FISHING

_____   Fishing rod

_____   Reel

_____   Fishing line

_____   Hooks

_____   Bobbers

_____   Flies

_____ Cord

_____ Tackle box

_____ Knife and/or small scissors

_____ Bait (though worms will do any old day!)

HUNTING

_____ Hunting Rifle

_____ Ammo

_____ Knife

_____ Rope

_____ Canvas

_____ Tarps

_____ Butcher paper

_____ Masking tape

_____ Hacksaw

_____ Snares

GARDENING

_____ Heirloom seeds (hybrid seeds are okay)

_____ Shovel

_____   Rake

_____   Hoe

_____   Trowel

_____   Clippers

_____   Hose

_____   Pots/buckets

_____   WD-40

_____   Duct tape

_____   String

_____   Sunblock

_____   Hat

_____   Gloves (many pair)

_____   Outdoor thermometer

_____   Plastic/garbage bags

• TIP: Get heirloom seeds to ensure the seeds from the fruits/vegetables you grow can be harvested to, in turn, grow more fruits and veggies the following year. Avoid genetically modified seeds.

• TIP: Learning to grow sprouts can provide a cheap, easy supply of vitamin-rich food.

☑**ACTION ITEM:** *Get the kids in a hunters' safety course.*

If your children are age 12 or older, you can enroll them in a hunters' safety course for a minimal fee in most areas. The instructors are typically part of that state's Fish and Wildlife Department, but private lessons are also available. Class participants are taught how to stalk prey, track, handle firearms safely, clean and skin an animal, and more.

Power and Transportation

You'll have to go old school if the electricity is gone. This leaves the option of either creating your own electricity or finding some alternative means of power. Getting your own wind turbines is probably out. Trees and the sun will help keep you warm and alive.

POWER

_____   Generator

_____   Spare generator parts

_____   Tanks of propane, diesel and gasoline

_____   Screwdrivers, wrenches, hammers—a full tool kit

_____   Solar panels/battery packs

_____   Chainsaw

_____   Extra saw chains

_____   Chainsaw oil

_____   Blade sharpener

_____   Gas tanks/can

_____   Axes

_____   Mauls

_____   Slitting wedges

_____   Hatchet

TRANSPORTATION

All it takes is a strong electromagnetic pulse used as a weapon, and virtually no vehicle on the road will start. Not your truck, not your ATV. What would you do if you were reduced to foot transportation only? How would you haul your firewood? Pack the hay you'd put up to your cattle?

_____   Wagons/carts (Just for fun we put them before the …)

_____   … Horses

_____   Bicycles

_____   Antique car—no computer/electronics inside? It'd start.

_____   Strollers—for infants and toddlers, but a lifesaver for you

Above and Beyond

If you've gone through this book, done the action items and checked off a lot of boxes, then you might start thinking about all the "extra" things you could do to prepare your secondary/bug-out or even your bug-in location. The possibilities are quite endless, so if you're overwhelmed from the rest of this little guide, shut it now and skip this chapter for a while. You can always come back to it later.

BUILD A BOMB SHELTER. If you have the time, location and the money, you might follow the instructions several hardcore preppers give: build yourself a bunker. Bomb shelters are often placed below the garage or basement of homes, far beneath the earth, but accessible from inside the house. Shelters can be constructed on site, or they can be transported nearly ready-made and installed there. Neither option is cheap. The ideal shelter will contain kitchen and bathroom areas, sleeping area, and a full stockroom of food and supplies that enable a family to live completely contained in these few rooms for weeks or sometimes even months. Shelters will be made of thick cement wall, sometimes lined with metal. Bomb-proof doors, multiple escape hatches and air filtration systems will be built in.

Contrary to popular belief, you can survive a nuclear blast. Of course, your odds improve the farther you are away from the detonation zone. Even if your area receives radioactive fallout, if you manage to stay put in a shelter for a couple weeks, the radiation dissipates. Keep potassium iodide tablets on hand in case you're exposed. Chem suits and radiation detection strips aren't bad ideas either.

COLLECT A LIBRARY. Imagine there are no classrooms, communication is limited, and besides—you're bored. After the sun goes down, what better way to give your kids an education that to have a full range of textbooks and fiction classics for them. Try to collect books on math, science, history, languages and whatever else you can find.

KEEP LIVESTOCK. If you have the space, cows, pigs, sheep, chickens, ducks, etc. would be lovely to own. You'll have nummies like meat, milk and eggs right at your fingertips. Raising livestock is complicated. You'll have to make sure you're able to keep them penned up on your property, and have the supplies for fencing. You'll have to make sure you have feed for them in the winter.

GROW YOUR OWN GRAINS. Again, if you have space, stockpile wheat, corn, barley or whatever floats your boat. Duplicate your gardening tools so you have spares. Invest in a good wheat mill/grinder. Doesn't your own flour or fresh cornmeal sound great?

LEARN TO MAKE SOAP. Well now, that's pretty self-explanatory, isn't it!?

START SEWING. It stands to reason that learning to stitch by hand and with a sewing machine might be wise moves. A few shelves full of needles, scissors, thread, buttons, zippers and fabric might serve you well.

STORE CLOTHING LIKE A CLOTHING STORE. You know how fast kids grow! You also know how fast an adult can wear through his boots and jeans when he's working outside everyday? If you have the space and the money, stack some shelves full of shirts, jeans, shoes, boots, etc. in each size your child will need as he or she grows. Extra adult-sized clothing may also be necessary in various sizes. Jeans, socks, underwear, boots and coats are extra important.

GO ON THE OFFENSIVE. Are you afraid of being raided? Buy books and take courses in self-defense. Learn to make booby traps. Invest in gas masks and body armor. If you want to go all *Red Dawn* to protect your home, learn how to first. If you're former military, you're one step ahead of the rest of us.

RELOAD. Rounds of ammo are cheaper when you reload them. Besides, factory ammo could be impossible to buy or barter for. You'll need shells, bullets, powder, scales and a full range of other reload supplies. Some folks set up entire rooms toward the pursuit of this hobby. Most likely, the corner of your basement would work just fine.

BECOME A TOYS R US PARENT. Kids outgrow their toys just like they outgrow their clothing. We would definitely file this idea away in the "luxury" category, but if you can put up some new toys for kids of all ages, the little ones will appreciate them in the future as they grow from little to not-so-little.

FILE THINGS AWAY. Collect all your vital, or formerly vital paperwork into one big envelope or file folder, and tuck it somewhere. (Keep it secret, keep it safe!) We're talking deeds, wills, birth certificates, bank statements, drivers' licenses, marriage certificates and the like. If you can make copies of your precious photos, do that as well. You might even make all these things in duplicate or triplicate and hide them in separate locations.

GO PIRATE AND BURY THE LOOT. If you find yourself with enough—or more supplies than you'll need—hide them away from you. Invest in air- and water-tight metal containers and bury extra ammo, dried foods or whatever have you in various locations that only you and your loved ones could find.

BECOME A BOTANIST. You might be in an area where the flora that grows wild can save your life. Study up on the local mushrooms, berries and weeds. Some could kill you. Some will sustain you. Some make for great medical treatments. Did you know the Native Americans used crushed wild strawberries as natural toothpaste? Now you do.

LEARN TO CAN. You'd be surprised how many people can their own fruits and veggies—even their own meat! You'll need bottles, tongs, lids, a large pot …

BECOME A BUG EXPERT. We weren't going to advise you to go eat bugs—unless you're desperate, then they're a great source of protein. Some bugs can also help your garden grow by chasing away pests. Knowing your bugs will also help you understand which spiders are poisonous and which disease symptoms probably came from that tick bite—then you can start medical treatment.

DRY YOUR FOOD. Invest in a solar or electrical food dehydrator. You'll be able to cut that venison into strips and make jerky, or the apples from your orchard into slices that can last a couple years.

GRADUATE TO ADVANCED PREPPER. After you've finished this working through this guide, beginning prepping will be too simple for you. There are prepper's networks, web sites and forums all over the Internet. More advanced guides are all over the marketplace. Remember, it's better to be thought of as a silly goose than to be a dead duck. Happy prepping!

www.ingramcontent.com/pod-product-compliance
Lightning Source LLC
Chambersburg PA
CBHW081022040426
42444CB00014B/3323